HANDBOOK OF
COMMON FOOT
PROBLEMS

HANDBOOK OF COMMON FOOT PROBLEMS

LAWRENCE B. HARKLESS, D.P.M.

Clinical Professor
Department of Orthopaedics/Podiatry Service
The University of Texas
Health Science Center at San Antonio
San Antonio, Texas

STEVEN M. KRYCH, D.P.M.

Assistant Professor
Department of Orthopaedics/Podiatry Service
The University of Texas
Health Science Center at San Antonio
San Antonio, Texas

CHURCHILL LIVINGSTONE
New York, Edinburgh, London, Melbourne

Library of Congress Cataloging-in-Publication Data

Harkless, Lawrence B.
   Handbook of common foot problems / Lawrence B.
Harkless, Steven M. Krych.
     p. cm.
   Includes bibliographical references.
   ISBN 0-443-08622-2
   1. Foot—Examination—Handbooks, manuals, etc.
2. Foot—Wounds and injuries—Handbooks, manuals,
etc. 3. Foot—Abnormalities—Handbooks, manuals,
etc. I. Krych, Steven M. II. Title.
   [DNLM: 1. Foot—abnormalities—handbooks.
2. Foot—injuries—handbooks. 3. Foot—
physiopathology—handbooks. 4. Foot
Diseases—diagnosis—handbooks.]
RD563.H29 1990
617.5'85—dc20
DNLM/DLC
for Library of Congress   90-1710
                                  CIP

Distributed in the United Kingdom by Churchill Livingstone,
Robert Stevenson House, 1–3 Baxter's Place, Leith Walk, Edinburgh
EH1 3AF, and by associated companies, branches, and
representatives throughout the world.

Accurate indications, adverse reactions, and dosage schedules for
drugs are provided in this book, but it is possible that they may
change. The reader is urged to review the package information data
of the manufacturers of the medications mentioned.

Acquisitions Editor: *Robert A. Hurley*
Copy Editor: *Kamely Dahir*
Production Designer: *Gloria Brown*
Production Supervisor: *Christina Hippeli*

Printed in the United States of America

First published in 1990

PREFACE

The impetus to write a book on common foot problems was generated by the interest of several family practice residents. They wanted a quick reference text on the foot to use while rotating on the Podiatry Service at the University of Texas Health Science Center at San Antonio.

The authors hope that the *Handbook of Common Foot Problems*, although not a textbook, will help the reader gain a better appreciation of foot problems, their evaluation, and normal function. The work-up section is problem oriented, designed to create a differential diagnosis list for appropriate treatment and referral. This book should be used to differentiate patient complaints into groups for better diagnosis of the etiology of the complaints. Each chapter has a section of suggested readings to research each area more completely. These lists are by no means all-inclusive, however, they may be used to acquire a literature review of specific foot problems.

We hope that this book will serve the needs of all the students, interns, residents, and practitioners who have a basic desire to learn how to evaluate, manage, and refer common foot problems.

Lawrence B. Harkless, D.P.M.
Steven M. Krych, D.P.M.

CONTENTS

1

HISTORY AND BASIC EXAMINATION OF THE FOOT

The foot is a complex and sensitive structure that is relegated to life within a shoe, which is often dictated by fashion. The foot's function is influenced by the shoe that is worn, as well as the surface the activity of the foot is performed on. The foot has two basic functions; first as a mobile adapter or shock absorber and second as a rigid lever or stable based for propulsion. These two functions require significantly different features. Age, flexibility, foot type, deformities, genetics, shoe gear, and the surfaces activities are performed on all affect the ability of the foot to perform these functions. The healthy foot, like the healthy body, needs proper nutrition, care, and environment to perform these functions. When deformity, trauma, or age-related changes do not allow the foot to function properly, symptoms are often associated. Most people wrongly assume that foot pain is a necessary component of life. This is not true and the pain can often be related to a specific event or activity. To find the etiology of the foot pain, a thorough history and physical examination is necessary.

The foot's physical examination consists of visualization, palpation, and knowledge of normal findings. It is of paramount importance to obtain an adequate history because the foot is often the recipient of neglectful treatment and overuse.

ANATOMY

Figures 1 and 2 represent the lateral, medial, and antero-posterior views of the foot illustrating its bony anatomy. The foot is comprised of 28 bones. Anatomically it can be broken down into the rearfoot, midfoot, and forefoot. The rearfoot consists of the talus and the calcaneus; the midfoot consists of the navicular, cuboid, and the three cuneiforms; and the forefoot consists of the metatarsals and phalanges (see Fig. 2). The arthrology of the foot consists of the distal interphalangeal (DIP) joints, the proximal interphalangeal (PIP) joints, hallux interphalangeal joint, the metatarsal phalangeal (MP) joints, Lisfranc's joint (tarsometatarsal joint), midtarsal joint (Chopart's joint), subtalar joint, and ankle joint. All of these joints are synovial joints. Figures 3, 4, 5, and 6 illustrate their motions and articulations. In the normal, healthy foot all joint range of motion (ROM) should be smooth without crepitus and without abrupt end. *Crepitus* is a crackling sound or feel when the joint is placed in motion. The figures illustrate normal ROMs. An overall understanding of the anatomy and the motions available at these joints helps the reader to appreciate the normal function of the foot and to better visualize pathologic function when presented with specific problems. The current literature contains several kinesiology textbooks for the reader to review the open and closed kinetic motions of these joints.

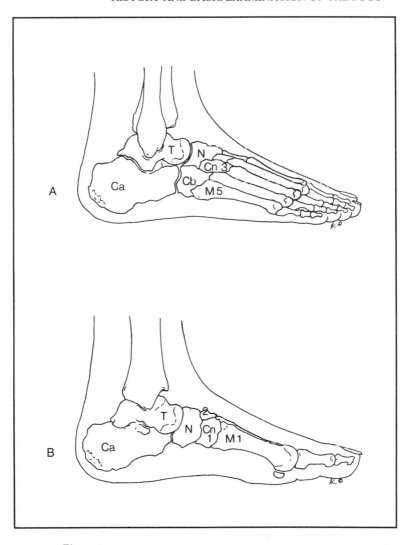

Figure 1
(A) Lateral view of the foot. (B) Medial view of the foot Ca, calcaneus;
Cb, cuboid; Cn, cuneiforms; M, metarsals; N, navicular; T, talus

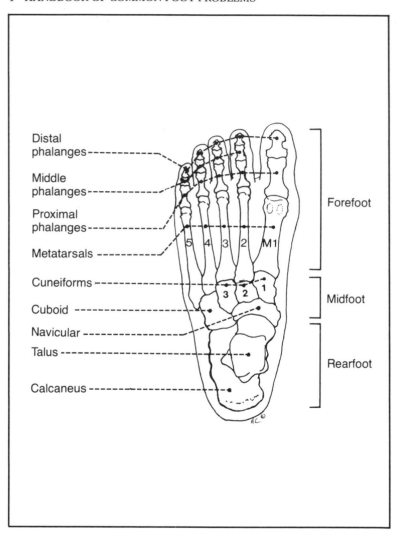

Figure 2
Anteroposterior view of the foot

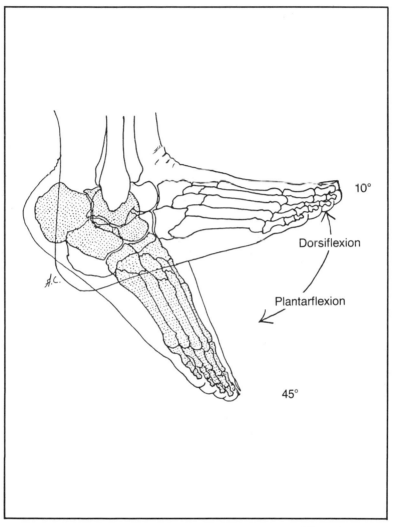

Figure 3
Ankle joint ROM

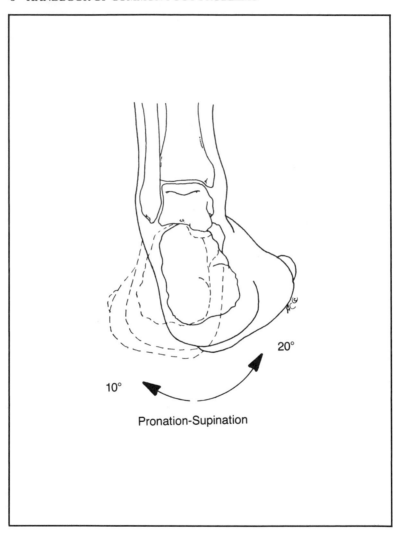

Figure 4
Primarily subtalar joint

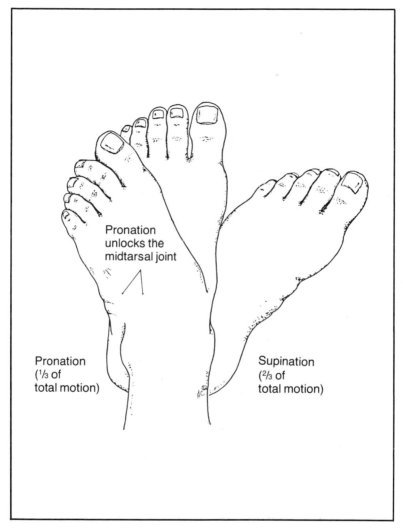

Figure 5
Primarily subtalar joint; secondarily midtarsal joint

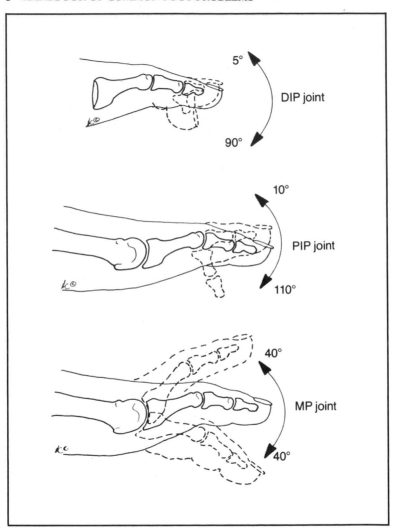

Figure 6
Digital ROM

EVALUATION

As with any patient, a standard format of chief complaint, history of present illness, past medical history, past surgical history, and sensitivities to drugs or treatments are necessary for a complete patient evaluation.

The history of the foot complaint is extremely important. In charting the complaint, we use the NLODCATS method in examining the patient (Table 1). All too often a patient will present after months of discomfort, and the physician will treat the generalized complaint rather than the etiology. Frequently these patients will have adjusted their gait and weight-bearing, which confuses the issue with a secondary overuse syndrome because of their compensation for the original pain. The NLODCATS method will help you isolate the problems.

Table 1. NLODCATS Method of Acquiring Foot Complaint's History

N = Nature of complaint
L = Location of complaint
O = Onset of symptoms
D = Duration of symptoms
C = Complicating factors (character of pain)
A = Aggravating factors
T = Previous treatments
S = Special considerations

PAIN

Pain is interpreted differently by individuals. While pain is a negative stimulus to most people, to others pain is considered a positive stimulus. An example may be an athlete who gets positive reinforcement from a work-out by the feeling experienced after full exertion. It is also well described that perception of pain is influenced by a person's psychologic state, fatigue, and the influences of secondary pain.

When examining a patient it is extremely important to have an idea of the types of pain associated with each injury. For example burning pain is often associated with nerve injury. Constant and unremitting burning pain can be associated with cellulitis, edema, a mass, or a constant pressure on a nerve. Burning pain aggravated by activity but relieved by rest or not felt when performing certain activities can often times be related to a localized impingement of a nerve either by local structures or by external forces. An example is sural nerve neuralgia caused by tight lace-up boots.

When a patient cannot describe their pain, associate it with aggravating or relieving factors, or localize the pain this should alert the examiner. The cause of this inability can be either a language barrier, a patient's mental handicap, psychologic influence, or a patient seeking secondary gain.

It is of extreme importance to determine the nature, location, and onset of the discomfort. The nature of the discomfort can be described as aching, burning, cramping, dull, sharp, throbbing, stabbing, etc. Often it is necessary to volunteer the adjectives to help the patient describe the nature of the discomfort. Frequently, the location is difficult to establish. A familiar scenario is a patient who simply waves a hand over the entire foot and states that it hurts. It is important to attempt to define the area of original discomfort because most of the time the generalized discomfort is secondary to compensation for the original complaint. Therefore, onset either by association with date, shoe gear, surface, or activity change is very important. It is important to specifically ask the patient what changes have taken place in their life or their daily activities prior to their symptoms. Examples might be a new job, a change in job role where they may be walking more, a change in their family life, or moving from a single story apartment to a two story apartment where there are multiple steps. An example of the nature of the pain could be a patient with diabetes complaining of nocturnal pain. The key differential questions are "Is the pain burning?; Is it sharp?; stabbing?; deep?; or superficial?" Generally, pain that is burning and superficial can be related to a neuropathic process. A sharp, stabbing, deep aching pain is often related to occlusive disease. The pattern of the pain should also be questioned "Does the patient notice the discomfort immediately upon attempting to fall asleep? Does the pain remain until the patient falls asleep or prevent the patient from falling asleep with no specific way to relieve the symptoms? Does the pain generally wake up the patient after having been asleep."

Neuropathic pain will usually involve a burning sensation and/or have a paresthetic character. It usually will keep the patient from falling asleep, and generally a sedative medication will allow the patient to fall asleep and these symptoms will subside. Ischemic pain allows the patient to fall asleep but it will often cause the patient to wake up as the evening progresses. The pain is frequently relieved by placing the limb in a dependent position by either standing, walking, or by hanging the foot over the end of the bed. This pain will have a deep, aching, sharp character aggravated by moderate amounts of activity. It is rarely relieved by pain medication. When presented with a patient with this type of complaint the clinician often elicits a similar type of complaint that is related to activity. Onset, duration, and course of the problem are always important especially if the patient can relate to any specific event. Always ask if the patient has changed any of their activities (e.g. job, weight, shoe gear). Pain associated with activity is often of a musculoskeletal origin as opposed to pain that is not associated with activity. For example, claudication pain occurs after walking a constant distance and tends to dissipate after a few minutes rest (i.e. window shopper's disease). Whereas, biomechanical fatigue or overuse pain will last much longer and may force the patient to a sitting position to completely rest the aching part. Also, a pattern of post-static dyskinesia is associated with a biomechanical abnormality. Plantar fasciitis or heel spur syndrome is a common cause of post-static dyskinesia associated with a biomechanical etiology. Clinical presentation usually includes pain upon arising in the morning that improves with activity; however, after sitting for awhile and resuming activity the pain recurs. In contrast, a tumor in the calcaneous may be painful regardless of activity level. The duration and cause of this discomfort is important in determining if the problem is becoming worse, staying the same, or improving. If the pain is not changing or if the patient cannot state whether there has been a change this should alert the clinician to secondary factors.

Subsequently there should be the determination of aggravating factors such as activity, weight-bearing, shoe gear, and surface, as previously mentioned. Previous treatments should be noted to avoid ineffective modalities and/or treatments that cause severe anxiety to the patient. This will allow previous beneficial modalities to be repeated.

Special considerations include prior trauma or surgery, patient's occupation, activity level, and whether the patient has any other physical or mental limitations that would necessitate adjustment of the treatment modalities. An example is an elderly patient with a bunion deformity who is bedridden versus a similar patient who is ambulatory. If you chose to treat the patients with accommodative devices, the bedridden patient would require quite a different device than the ambulatory patient.

SUGGESTED READINGS

Bates B: A Guide to Physical Examination and History Taking. 4th Ed. JB Lippincott, Philadelphia, 1987

Lacote M, Chevailier AM, Miranda A et al: Clinical Evaluation of Muscle Function. 2nd Ed. Churchill Livingstone, Edinburgh, 1987

McGlamry ED: Fundamentals of Foot Surgery. Williams & Wilkins, Baltimore, 1987

Post M: Physical Examination of the Musculo-Skeletal System. Yearbook Medical Publishers, Chicago, 1987

Seidel HM, Ball JW, Dains JE, Benedict GW: Mosby's Guide to Physical Examination. CV Mosby, St. Louis, 1987

2

PHYSICAL EXAMINATION IN SPECIFIC SYSTEMS

A physical examination requires that the examiner fully understand the definition of a normal foot. The normal foot is a rectus foot type that has supple, flexible skin with no areas of hyperpigmentation. The joint ROM for all joints is supple and pain free with *all* muscles having 5/5 muscle strength. Pulses are palpable and strong without bounding, and the capillary refill time is less than 3 seconds to each digit. The deep tendon reflexes are at least 3/5 without being hyper-reflexive and there is intact sensation and proprioception. During gait the foot exhibits normal sequential weight-bearing without ROM extremes.

A standard examination includes observational, vascular, dermatologic, neurologic, musculoskeletal, and gait testing. It should first focus on the system related to the chief complaint.

OBSERVATION

Note the overall appearance of the patient, affect, gait, height, weight, posture, hygiene, and shoe gear. Observe the relative ease or difficulty with which they get into the treatment chair and their strength and flexibility when unlacing and removing shoes. This will influence the treatment plan toward modifications if limitations exist. Look for gross deformity, discoloration, open wounds, venous distension, swelling, and any contours which vary from normal anatomy. These findings will contribute to a more rapid and complete diagnosis, as well as cue the examiner to specific questions about the patient's past medical history.

VASCULAR EXAMINATION

The vascular examinations consists of palpating and grading the blood supply to the foot at the popliteal, dorsalis pedis, and posterior tibial arteries. This is performed using the sensitive fat pad of the finger tips. (Fig. 7 and 8, Table 2). Care should be taken to note differences between the pulses. Signs and symptoms consistent with a significant vascular history warrant appropriate vascular laboratory workup (Table 3). The subpapillary venous plexus filling-time is also used to determine the status of the smaller vessels. Normal filling-time is approximately 3 to 4 seconds. This is performed with the foot at the level of the heart, blanching the distal digital skin, and noticing the time it takes for the digital skin to return to normal color. The Trendelenburg test of the lower extremities is used to evaluate valvular insufficiency of the venous system. In patients with vascular disease Doppler ultrasound and infrared-venous plethysmography are quick, inex-

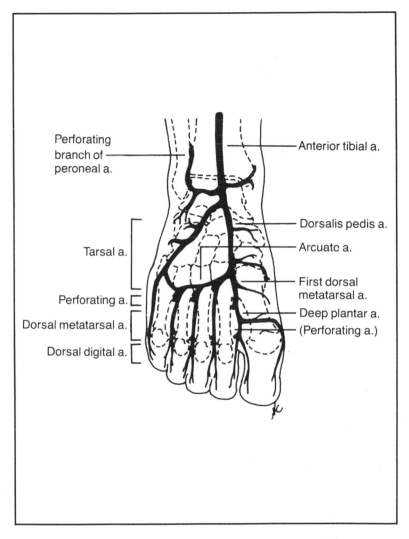

Perforating branch of peroneal a.

Anterior tibial a.

Dorsalis pedis a.

Arcuate a.

Tarsal a.

First dorsal metatarsal a.

Perforating a.

Deep plantar a.

Dorsal metatarsal a.

(Perforating a.)

Dorsal digital a.

Figure 7
Dorsal arteries

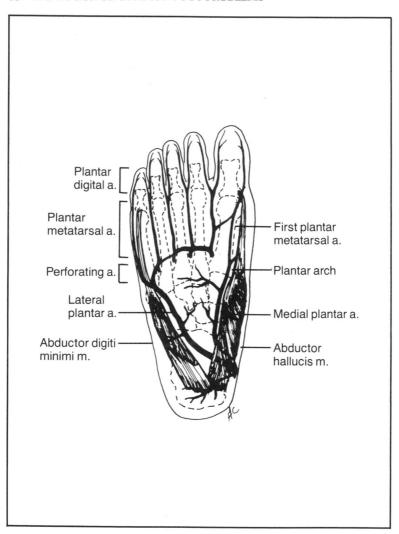

Figure 8
Plantar arteries

Table 2. Pulses

0	= Nonpalpable
+1	= Palpable but weak
+2	= Strong and regular
+3	= Normal
+4	– Bounding

Table 3. Signs and Symptoms of Peripheral Vascular Disease

Loss of hair on the foot or toes
Shiny or xerotic appearance of the skin
Dystrophic nail changes
Painful nails without clinical signs of infection
Absent pulses
Delayed capillary refill time and blanching of skin
  on elevation
Atrophy of subcutaneous tissues of toes
Blanching of skin over bony prominences
Intermittent claudication
Noctural pain relieved with dependency

pensive office tests. These tests can provide information as to the extent of vascular disease and allow for a more timely referral and treatment.

DERMATOLOGIC EXAMINATION

If the patient presents with a lesion, the ability to describe it is most important in making the diagnosis. Common dermatologic nomenclature should be used. Lesions should be described as primary or secondary (Table 4). Observation should be made as to color, vascularity, type of lesion, edema, moisture, temperature, texture, mobility, rash, scarring, corns and calluses, and

Table 4. Primary and Secondary Dermatologic Lesions

Primary	Secondary
Macule	Scales
Papule	Crusts
Nodule	Excoriations
Vesicle	Fissures
Patch	Ulcers
Plaque	Scars
Tumor	Lichenification
Bullae	
Pustules	
Petechiae	
Purpura	

hygiene. The nails should be examined for presence, color, shape, and thickness. Determination should also be made of the pedal hair and its pattern of distribution and the level of loss. Many systemic diseases show early signs in the skin that can help confirm diagnosis. An example is the presentation of erythematous, raised plaques on the extensor skin combined with joint pain and pitted nails which may lead the examiner to a differential diagnosis including psoriasis.

NEUROLOGIC EXAMINATION

A neurologic examination is important in patients with a history consistent with neurologic etiology, chronic disease, or trauma. Examination should consist of assessment of the patellar and Achilles deep tendon reflexes, proprioception, and sharp/dull, temperature, and vibratory sensation. In diabetic patients, muscle

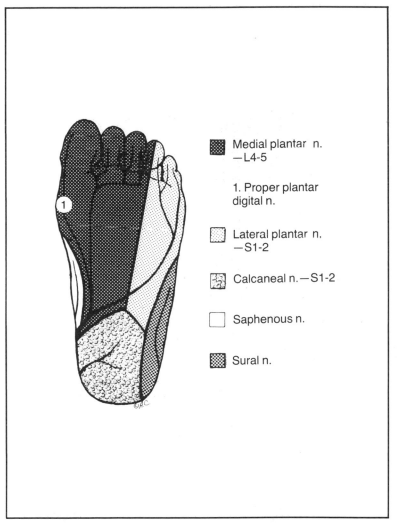

Figure 9
Cutaneous innervation—plantar aspect

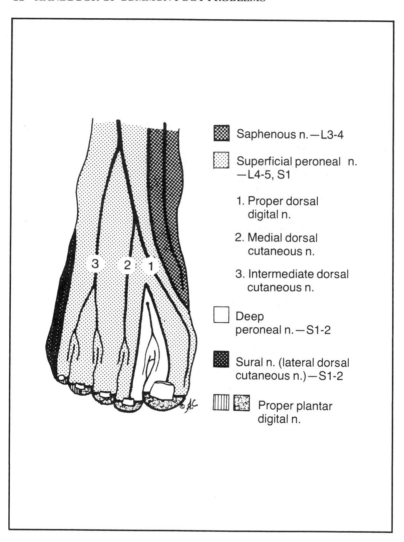

Figure 10
Cutaneous innervation—dorsal aspect

Table 5. Signs and Symptoms of Neuropathy in the Foot of the Diabetic Patient

Noctural pain not allowing the patient to fall asleep

Paresthesia, hypoesthesia/hyperasthesia early in the course of the disease with a patchy distribution; late in the course of the disease with a stocking pattern

Hemorrhage within a callus or subungually, associated with no pain and no recollection of trauma

Evidence of injury without patient recollection

Patient wearing improperly fitted shoes

Loss of deep tendon reflexes and vibratory, pressure, temperature, and position sense

Changes in the shape of the foot, pointing of the toes, increase or decrease in arch height

Radiographic signs of osteolysis, Charcot changes, or demineralization

Drop foot gait, slapping type gait, or wide base gait

Intrinsic muscular atrophy

Decubitus ulceration

function and assessment of the ability to use the muscles effectively in gait may provide important clues to neurologic deficit. The Semmes-Weinstein monofilament will help quantify the level of protective sensation. In order to properly evaluate trauma including lacerations and gunshot wounds, it is always important to understand the dermatomal patterns as well as the anatomic distribution of the nerves to the foot (Fig. 9 and 10, Table 5). If a nerve is injured a specific pattern is seen and should be mapped out on the foot and illustrated in the patient's chart.

MUSCULOSKELETAL EXAMINATION

The musculoskeletal examination consists of establishing function and strength of the foot muscles. Figures 11, 12, and 13 show the course of the muscles listed in

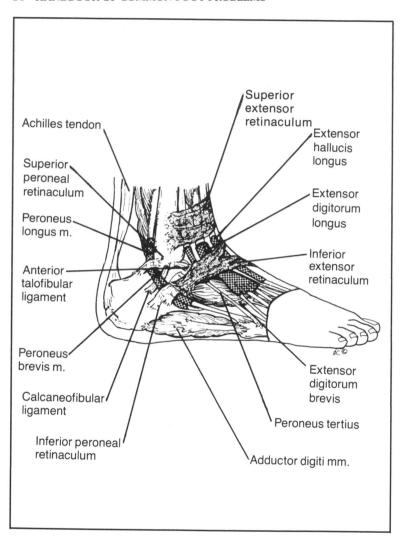

Figure 11
Tendons—lateral view

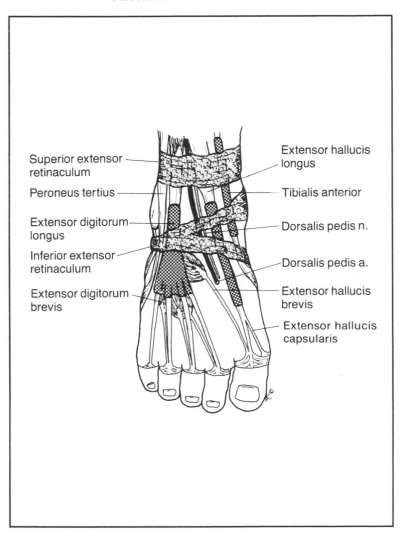

Figure 12
Tendons—dorsal view

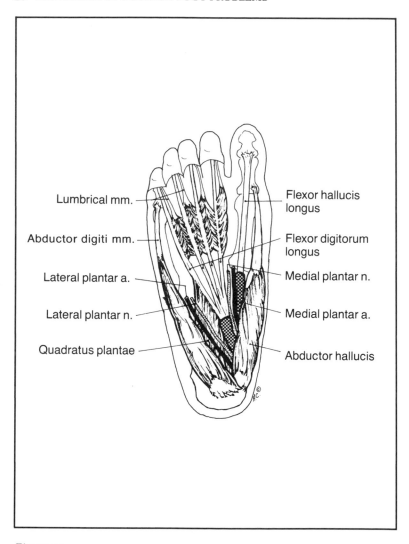

Figure 13
Tendons—plantar view

Table 6. Intrinsic Musculature

Extensor digitorum brevis —only
    intrinsic muscle on the dorsum
Flexor digitorum brevis
FDQB
FDH
Abductus hallucis
Adductus hallucis
Quadratus plantae
Lumbricals
Plantar interossei 3
Dorsal interossei 4

Tables 6 and 7 along with their insertions. This is extremely important in determining injuries that would involve a tendon or a tendon sheath, as well as determining progression of peripheral neuropathy in patients with diabetes. Standard muscle grading criteria are used (Table 8). With practice, an examiner should be able to isolate most of the individual muscles of the foot. A simple cursory way to evaluate muscle strength is to

Table 7. Extrinsic Musculature

Gastrocnemius
Soleus
Plantaris
Tibialis anterior
Extensor digitorum longus
Extensor hallucis longus
Peroneus longus
Peroneus brevis
Peroneus tertius
Flexor digitorum longus
Flexor hallucis longus
Posterior tibial

Table 8. Muscle Grading

0 = No motion, no evidence of contraction
1 = Contraction, no movement without gravity
2 = Full motion with gravity
3 = Full motion against gravity
4 = Full motion, can be resisted by examiner
5 = Full motion, motion without signs of fatigue

have the patient stand on his toes, heels, inside of feet, and outside of feet during gait. Inability to perform these functions is indicative of a musculoskeletal abnormality.

GAIT EXAMINATION

Gait examination is facilitated with a 20-foot long, well lit hallway. Begin the examination by noticing the change in the shape of the foot from non-weight-bearing to weight-bearing, including the medial talar bulge, the spreading of the metatarsals, and the relationship of the tendons. Have the patient walk up and down the hallway at their usual rate of speed. Note the overall posture of the patient, head and neck, shoulder heights, arm swing, and hip height, as well as hip rotation, patellar height, knee flexion in swing, and ankle motion. Observe the relationship of the bisection of the tibia to the ground and the bisection of the calcaneous to the ground. Now note the alignment of the rearfoot to the forefoot and the forefoot to the toes. With the patient walking notice if the heel strikes the ground inverted, perpendicular, or everted, and if the heel moves as the patient's weight is transferred from the heel to the forefoot. Next watch the foot pronate as the weight transfers from the rearfoot to the forefoot to absorb shock and then watch as the arch begins to rise as weight is taken off the heel and transferred to the ball of the foot and toes. Note the position of the toes, the bulging of the tendons, and the position of the foot as it is lifted off the ground for the swing phase of gait. It is important to observe the patient at different rates of speed to help determine if the proper muscles are firing at the proper times. When excessive pronation or inadequate pronation are present this can indicate specific clinical problems. During this examination have the patient stand on his toes, heels, and outside of foot to confirm functional muscle activity.

SUGGESTED READINGS

Bates B: A Guide to Physical Examination and History Taking. 4th Ed. JB Lippincott, Philadelphia, 1987

Lacote M, Chevailer AM, Miranda A et al: Clinical Evaluation of Muscle Function. 2nd Ed. Churchill Livingstone, Edinburgh, 1987

McGlamry ED: Fundamentals of Foot Surgery. William & Wilkins, Baltimore, 1987

Post M: Physical Examination of the Musculo-Skeletal System. Yearbook Medical Publishers, Chicago, 1987

Seidel HM, Ball JW, Dains JE, Benedict GW: Mosby's Guide to Physical Examination. CV Mosby, St. Louis, 1987

3

DERMATOLOGY

The integument is the single largest organ of the body and reflects the overall condition of the body. Plantar, like palmar, skin significantly differs from the rest of the skin of the body.

The plantar skin of the foot is unique in several ways. It is markedly thickened, and although eccrine glands are numerous, apocrine glands, sebaceous glands, and hair follicles are absent. Most people enclose their feet in synthetic stockings or shoes for fashion rather than function. This unique environment is often times the etiology of the presenting complaint.

CORNS AND CALLUSES

Neglected corns and calluses can be symptomatic. Corns are of two basic types and are located on the digits. Heloma durum (hard corns) are found on the tops, tips, and sides of the toes, and Heloma molle (soft corns) are found in the web spaces, primarily the fourth. The etiology of corns is irritation of the overlying skin by one or a combination of the following: (1) shoe gear over a bony prominence, (2) two adjacent bony surfaces, or (3) distal bone and the ground.

Calluses can be the result of improper weight-bearing, malfunctioning eccrine glands, or heredity. A callus is an area of thick hyperkeratotic skin, with continuous skin lines on the bottom of the foot. A wart is commonly mistaken for a callus. Warts can be identified by the presence of a distinct capsule, loss of skin lines, and pinpoint bleeding upon debridement. Warts tend to exhibit more tenderness to direct palpation than do calluses. The etiology of a wart is viral, and therefore a cure is impossible.

Hereditary calluses can be diffentiated from biomechanical lesions by their presence in non-weight-bearing areas, presence in childhood, and their often concomitant involvement of the palmar and plantar skin. A history of a parent or relative having a similar distribution can usually be elicited.

Porokeratosis plantaris discreta, a type of plantar callus, is believed to be associated with malfunctioning eccrine glands. This can be differentiated from a callus or wart by presence of a white central nucleus after debridement, extreme pain with side-to-side pressure "chandelier sign," the presence of hyperhidrosis, and mycotic nails. Hyperhidrosis may be exhibited by a yellowing of plantar calluses, thickened odiferous nails, chronic tinea pedis, and dyshidrotic eczema, even in the absence of a moist, sweaty foot at the time of examination. This lesion is one of the most painful on the foot with a high degree of recurrence following excision.

The most common dermatologic problem in the foot is tinea pedis of which there are two basic types: (1) the acute, pruritic, vesicular, and (2) the chronic scaling. Acute tinea can often be mistaken for dyshidrotic eczema and candida. Acute tinea may be complicated by bacterial infection secondary to eczematization by the itch-scratch cycle. Generally candida is confined to the intertriginous areas of the foot, usually the web spaces, and diagnosis can be confirmed by culture. History is important in diagnosis of dyshidrosis. Patients are usually anxious and nervous with stress being the precipitating factor in lesion development. Pompholyx or dyshidrotic eczema is characterized by deep seated vesicles, with thick roofed blebs on a nonerythematous base that heal by desquamation. Evidence of eczema is often seen on other body parts such as the hands, elbows, and scalp. All of the above can become secondarily infected, and this will alter the clinical presentation. The bacterial infection should be treated before the underlying dermatologic problem. Acute pruritic tinea presents with multiple thin roofed blebs, peripheral erythema, pruritus, thin clear to whitish drainage, and is usually confined to intertriginous and plantar skin. Chronic scaling tinea generally has a moccasin distribution of the plantar foot with thin roofed dry blebs with little or no erythema or pruritus. Both types of tinea can be associated with fungal toenail involvement.

INGROWN TOENAILS

An ingrown toenail is a common problem and usually presents in three distinct populations, the neonate, adolescent, and elderly. Table 9 lists nail terminology.

The clinical presentation in the neonate is due to hypertrophy of the ungual labia of the digits with a very broad flat nail plate. The neonate will be presented because of nonresolution of the erythema and edema. These generally do not present with granuloma; however, they may have a serous drainage.

The ingrown nail is seen most commonly in the ado-

Table 9. Nail Terminology

Koilonychia: spoon nail, concave shape

Onycholysis: separation of the nail from the nailbed distally toward proximally

Onychomadesis: separation of the nail plate from the nailbed proximally toward distally

Leukonychia: whitening of the nail plate

Paronychia: inflammation of skin along the nail margins

Onychia: inflammation of the nailbed

Anonychia: absence of nail

Onychauxis: hypertrophy of the nail

Onychogryphosis: a deformed overgrowth of the nail plate producing a hook or incurvation

Onychocryptosis: incurvation of the nail borders into the nail grooves

Onychomycosis: fungal infection of the nail

lescent. In this group it often presents in the hallux with an incurvated nail plate, granulation tissue, and hypertrophic nail borders. Frequently the toe shows signs of drainage and a foul odor. The etiology is a foreign body reaction between the nail plate and the soft tissue exacerbated by shoe pressure. There is often periungual edema, erythema, hypertrophy of the periungual tissue, and drainage. If no systemic signs of infection are present and there is no complicating disease process, the ingrown nail can be treated as a foreign body. The offending border of nail should be removed permanently to prevent regrowth. The clinician should always be aware of the close proximity of the underlying phalanx and rule out bone involvement especially in chronic cases or cases which have been previously treated.

In the elderly, the ingrown nail is associated with an incurvated nail or hypertrophic changes of the nail as a result of onychomycosis or decreasing blood supply.

Great care should be taken when treating the ingrown nail of the elderly. Often the nail plate is adhered to the nailbed further distally than normal. With the age-related changes of vision and flexibility, the toenails are often neglected and become hypertrophied. When the physical examination reveals minimal erythema, edema, nonpalpable pulses, and severe discomfort with light touch, a vascular origin should be considered. An appropriate vascular evaluation is indicated before definitive treatment. The etiology of the pain is usually due to the plate of the nail irritating a marginally viable nailbed.

ONYCHOMYCOSIS

Fungal involvement of the nail plate begins distally with a separating of the nail plate from the nailbed. This will usually progress to involve the entire nailbed and matrix. These nails are almost always thickened, yellow to golden brown in color, and separated from the nailbed. When the fungal involvement includes the matrix the nail will become dystrophic and can grow in almost any shape or direction. These nails are usually asymptomatic unless elongated or irritated by tight shoes. They can become a risk area when the patient has decreased protective sensation and is therefore unaware of the abnormal pressure. Clinically this may be seen as a subungual hematoma in the absence of any related history of trauma. The distal loosening of the nail plate also creates a longer lever arm of the nail that causes symptoms at the proximal nailbed due to motion of the nail plate.

Oftentimes the pattern of involvement of onychomycosis includes only the hallux and the fifth toe. This presentation has been related to the trauma which allows the fungus to invade the nailbed. With time the fungus will progress to involve all the nails.

DYSTROPHIC NAILS

Dystrophic nails can be differentiated from the fungal nails by the nail's adherence to the nailbed and its incurvated or pincer growth pattern. Dystrophic nails are most often seen in the middle-aged to geriatric patient and can be very painful. Care should be taken when reducing these nails because the nailbed is adhered to the nail plate much further distally than the normal nail. If the patient has some form of peripheral vascular disease, overzealous reduction of the nail and nailbed can lead to an infected ischemic wound. Earlier these nails may appear similar to a club nail.

COMBINATION MYCOTIC AND DYSTROPHIC NAILS

The combination of mycotic and dystrophic nails are seen in the geriatric population and can be difficult to treat because of the associated pain and the likelihood of infection. Permanent removal of the nail is the best treatment provided circulation is adequate for healing.

Many other systemic and local diseases are expressed in the skin of the foot. Transverse lines of the nails are seen frequently following a severe illness. The reader is advised to review other textbooks for a more in-depth explanation of pedal dermatologic patterns.

SUGGESTED READINGS

Levy LA, Hetherington VJ: Principles and Practice of Podiatric Medicine. Churchill Livingstone, New York, 1990

McCarthy DJ: Podiatric Dermatology. Williams & Wilkins, Baltimore, 1986

Yale I: Podiatric Medicine. 2nd Ed. Williams & Wilkins, Baltimore, 1980

4

SOFT TISSUE INJURIES

Because of the foot's anatomic location it is often the recipient of trauma. This chapter reviews the more common soft tissue injuries. It is assumed that tetanus immunization has been reviewed and appropriate steps have been taken to update the patient's immunization.

PUNCTURE WOUNDS

Puncture wounds can have serious sequelae; therefore a careful history of the event is very important in determining the depth of the wound as well as the likelihood of a foreign body being present. Radiographs are important because puncture wounds involving bone or joints, foreign bodies, or gas are a surgical emergency and must be opened, drained, and any involved tissue debrided. Foreign bodies such as toothpicks, glass, needle and thread, BB, or rubber have all been found in wounds. Some foreign bodies cannot be visualized radiographically; therefore even innocuous appearing wounds deserve complete evaluation, including cleansing and debridement of the puncture tract (Fig. 14 and 15). When the puncture wound is in close proximity to a bone or joint, exploration of the wound will help determine

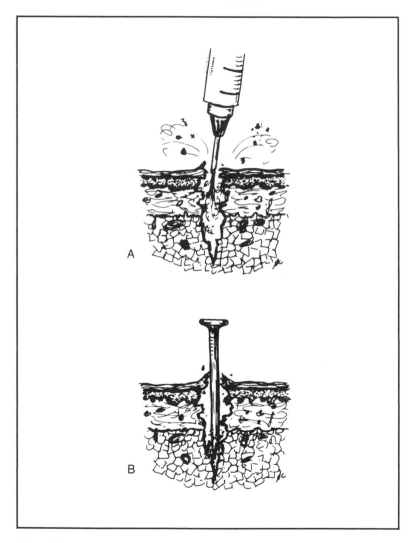

Figure 14
(A) Wound lavage. (B) Puncture wound

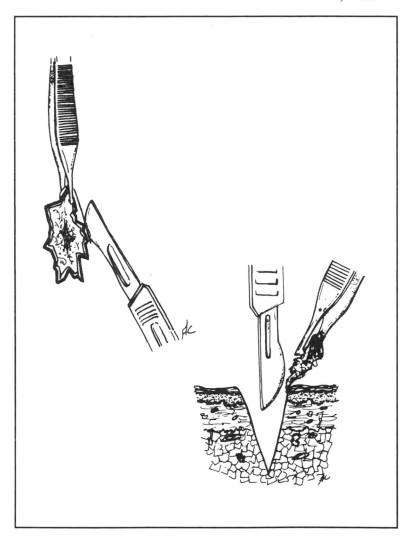

Figure 15
Surgical debridement of puncture site

bone or joint involvement. Most wounds that progress to deep infection do so because of inadequate debridement. Late sequelae of puncture wounds are foreign body or epidermal inclusion cysts. These usually present after some type of irritation to the area and present as localized, painful masses that are solid, intra-epidermal, nonmovable, nontransluminable, and non-pulsatile.

CRUSH WOUNDS

Crush injury to the foot is seen frequently. With all crush wounds soft tissue involvement as well as tissue viability must be assessed, and in this regard neurologic and vascular examinations are of priority. The dorsum of the foot has very thin tissue covering the bone and it is not unusual to have a resultant vasculitic episode or neurapraxia secondary to a crush injury. Definitive treatment should be delayed until the extent of the tissue damage, which often times takes several days, is determined. If the injury involves the nail with subungual hemorrhage as well as fracture, these injuries should be treated as open fractures. Radiographs will determine the osseous involvement. Injuries not complicated by bony involvement are best treated with drainage of the hematoma, sterile dressing, and immobilization. An option to evaluate the area of injury is to trace the area of erythema on presentation and to observe for any changes in size during the next 24 to 48 hours. The clinician should always be cautious of compartment syndromes when treating this type of injury. Unremitting pain and distal ischemia are positive clinical signs for a compartment syndrome. A late complication of such injuries is fibrosis of the overlying soft tissues and contracture; therefore, both active and passive physical therapy exercises are necessary.

LACERATIONS

It is very important to determine the cause of a laceration and to obtain a complete history from the patient. A laceration occurring while using a clean knife presents a very different wound than a laceration with a dirty knife because of the debris introduced into the wound. Prior to selecting a mode of repair, it is important to accurately determine the vascular and neural involvement on any laceration that transects the foot. While a laceration to the lateral foot may be sutured and heal uneventfully, an unrecognized sural nerve deficit may lead to future neuropathic complications over the prominent fifth metatarsal head. Lacerations should be assumed to be contaminated until cultures prove otherwise. It is important to be aware of the "golden rule" of wound closure—if there is any question of the wound being dirty, closure should be delayed until proper antibiosis and granulation tissue are present.

SPRAINS AND STRAINS

The ankle is the most commonly injured part of the foot, but is often not evaluated adequately. As in any injury, it is very important to establish the mechanism of injury. The most common injury of the ankle is the lateral ankle sprain or supination injury of the ankle. This occurs when the ankle and foot are plantarflexed. There is instability of the ankle mortice due to the shape of the talus. This plantarflexion places increased stress on the anterior talofibular ligament. Other ligaments most commonly injured in an ankle sprain include the calcaneofibular, posterior talofibular, posterior tibiofibular syndesmosis, and deltoid ligaments of the medial ankle (Figs. 16, 17, 18). Radiographic observation is necessary to rule out bony involvement. Examination of the injured ankle begins by examining the uninjured ankle. This is because there is often pain and swelling associated with the injury, as well as apprehension and splinting by the patient. While the patient is supine and the foot is at 90 degrees to the leg, palpate the anterior central ankle joint and begin palpating laterally around the ankle joint. The first structure you come to will be the long extensor tendon; just lateral to this is the anterior talofibular ligament at the level of the anterior distal fibula and the talar neck. The calcaneofibular ligament will be found at the distal most aspect of the fibula and can be felt by inverting the ankle causing the ligament to be taut. This can be difficult due to the overlying peroneal tendons and sheath. Next the posterior talofibular ligament at the distal posterior aspect of the fibula and the posterior aspect of the talus can be palpated. Palpate posteriorly and medially to determine involvement of the posterior talofibular syndesmosis and the deltoid ligament. Place the ankle through plantarflexion, and dorsiflexion to determine the quality and degree of motion. Then with the foot plantarflexed to the leg, place an inversion force on the ankle; this will help determine the motion available when the anterior talofibular ligament is under stress. To stress the calcaneofibular ligament, place the foot at 90 degrees to the leg and put inversion stress on the ankle. The anterior

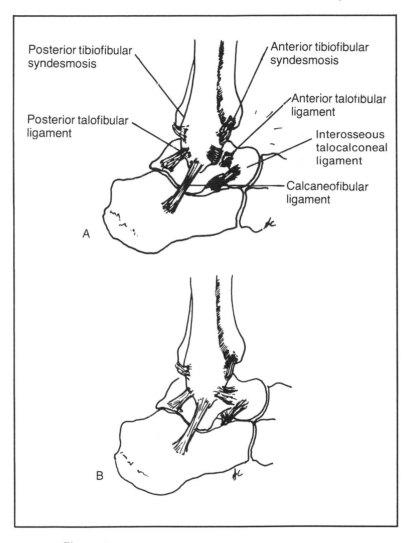

Figure 16
(A) Ruptured anterior talofibular ligament. (B) Normal lateral ligament

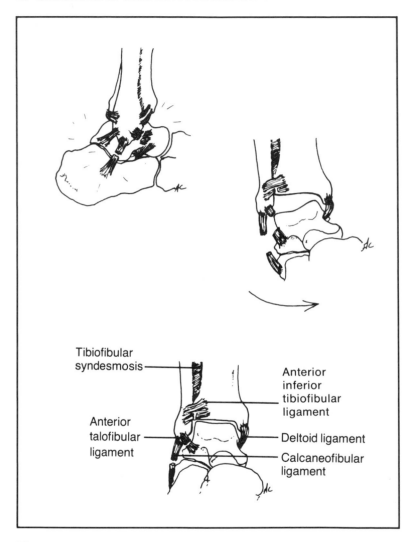

Figure 17
Anatomy of soft tissue ankle injuries

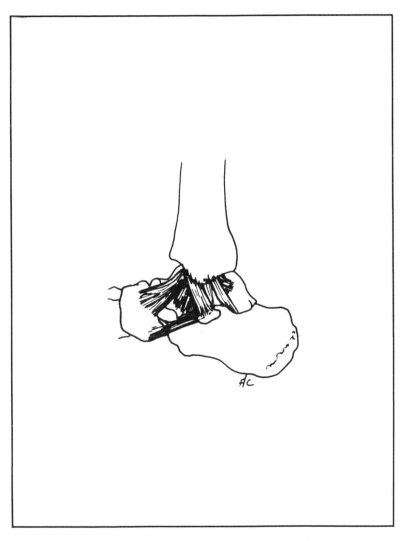

Figure 18
Deltoid ligaments

and posterior drawer test are used to differentiate rupture and strain of the anterior talofibular ligament. The inversion stress test with the foot at 90 degrees to the leg will assess the calcaneofibular ligament. The most significant inequalities of available inversion found during the inversion stress test will usually indicate combined injury of both the anterior talofibular and the calcaneofibular ligaments. Examination should always include the peroneus brevis insertion at the base of the fifth metatarsal where an avulsion fracture may be overlooked. Now examine the injured ankle. Readers are encouraged to review the vast amount of literature available on ankle evaluation and to create for themselves a standard ankle evaluation technique.

SUGGESTED READINGS

Heckman JD: New Techniques in Management of Foot Trauma. Clin Orthop 240:105, 1989

Scurran BL: Foot and Ankle Trauma. Churchill Livingstone, New York, 1989

5

COMMON BONE INJURIES

Fractures of the foot are classified by the location, type of fracture line, deformity, stability, and whether it is an open or closed injury (Figs. 19 and 20). All fractures that are open require surgical intervention and intravenous antibiotics. Generally, deformity, edema, and pain are the presenting complaints. Patients will commonly present 24 to 48 hours after an injury, thus, complicating immobilization due to edema. Vascular and neurologic function must be assessed before any treatment is begun. In these cases it is necessary to immobilize the part and apply a compressive dressing to mobilize the edema before casting. Radiographs will usually show a fracture when at least three different views of the involved part are taken (see Figs. 19 and 20). In the case of stress fractures a bone scan immediately or repeat radiography approximately 2 weeks after injury will confirm a clinical diagnosis. Any fractures involving a joint or the insertion of a tendon will require rigid immobilization and occasionally surgical intervention. These measures must also consider the long-term plan for eventual rehabilitation, restoration of strength, motion, and overall function.

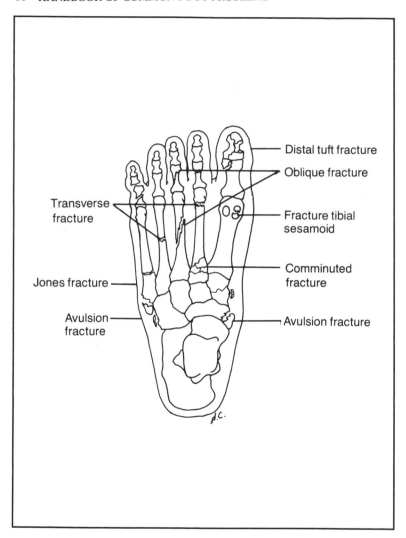

Figure 19
Common fractures of the foot seen on an anteroposterior radiograph

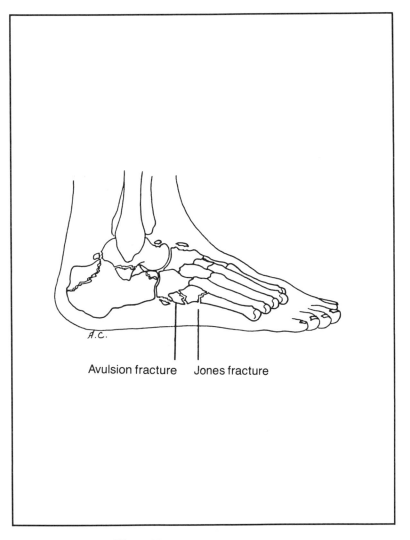

Figure 20
Common fractures of the foot seen on a lateral radiograph

JONES FRACTURE

The Jones fracture is a fracture of the proximal shaft of the fifth metatarsal distal to the tuberosity. This fracture is known to proceed to nonunion if improperly treated. It is often associated with an inversion or dorsiflexion injury. If nondisplaced, the patient should be treated in a cast for 6 to 8 weeks. After 8 weeks of casting radiographs should be taken to evaluate healing. If healing is not present, immobilization should be continued up to 6 months. After 6 months of treatment with no evidence of healing an open reduction and internal fixation (ORIF) should be performed.

AVULSION FRACTURE OF THE BASE OF THE FIFTH METATARSAL

This fracture can be confused with the Jones fracture; however, an avulsion fracture *only* involves the insertion of the peroneus brevis. This fracture is often associated with a lateral ankle injury. Oftentimes a fracture can appear similar to the accessory ossicle, os vesalianum.

HALLUX SESAMOID FRACTURES

The diagnosis of a sesamoid fracture can be elusive. Often a patient will present with an insidious onset of pain and swelling under the great toe joint with no history of trauma. The differential diagnosis should include stress fracture, sesamoiditis, and flexor tendonitis. Radiographs will confirm the diagnosis of a stress fracture; however, a bipartite or tripartite sesamoid can radiographically appear the same as a fracture. It is often necessary to obtain bilateral views to rule out bipartite or tripartite sesamoids since they occur bilaterally. It is possible to have a bipartite sesamoid with inflammation secondary to weight-bearing stress mimicking a fracture. A diagnosis of sesamoiditis is present when pain is elicited upon palpation of either sesamoid without evidence of fracture. Flexor tendonitis is diagnosed when pain is elicited at the plantar aspect of the neck of the first metatarsal with active flexion of the great toe. An axial sesamoidal view should be taken if sesamoid pathology is suspected. This can also be helpful in differentiating arthritis versus osteochondritis of the sesamoid. These fractures are notoriously slow healers because of their location in the tendon sheath and the pull of the flexor hallucis brevis, which is poorly vascularized and difficult to immobilize necessitating removal. When reasonable conservative therapy treatment fails sesamoidectomy is indicated.

METATARSAL FRACTURES

Fractures involving the metatarsals should be evaluated for sagittal or transverse plane deformity. Deformity significant enough to alter the weight-bearing function of the metatarsals should be reduced. Metatarsal fractures can be slow healing due to weight-bearing stresses. Depending on the patient's compliance, these fractures should be immobilized in a surgical shoe or cast to assure proper healing.

GROWTH PLATES VERSUS FRACTURES

When a child presents with an injury, radiographs of the opposite nontraumatized limb can help determine if a child has a Salter type fracture. Care should be taken in making this assessment with consultation as needed to avoid misdiagnosis of a Salter injury that can lead to growth disturbances and deformity if not treated properly. In a Salter type injury the parents should be made aware of the possibility of a growth disturbance at the time of diagnosis.

TUFT FRACTURES

Tuft fractures are often associated with subungual hematomas. The interphalangeal (IP) joint is often involved and will become stiff. Clinical examination should place all potentially involved joints through a full ROM to identify pathology.

ACCESSORY OSSICLES

The accessory bones are often confused with fractures. Bilateral occurrence, smooth contours, and lucency between ossicles help differentiate bipartite ossicles from fractures (Figs. 21 and 22).

Because of the foot's end-organ status as well as weight-bearing responsibilities, it is to be expected that swelling and discomfort remain for longer periods of time than with the upper extremity.

In a patient that complains of constant pain the clinician should be aware of the possibility of reflex sympa-

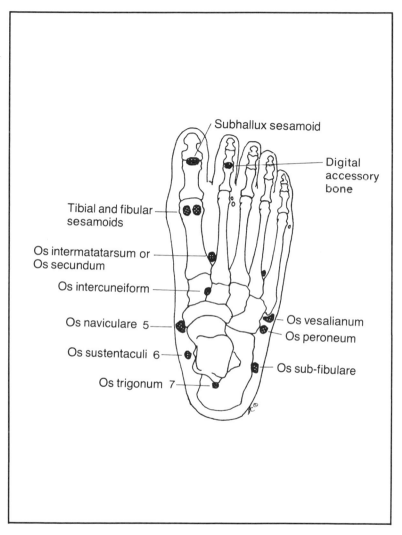

Figure 21
Accessory bones (anteroposterior view)

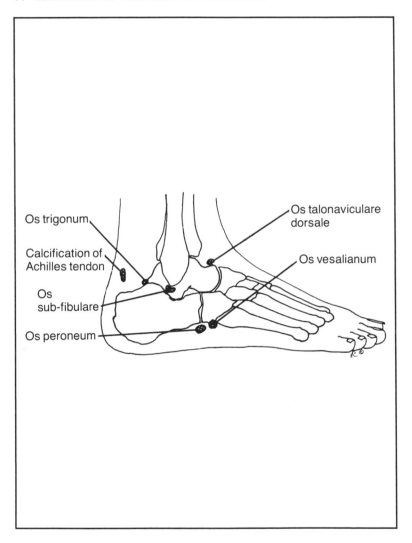

Figure 22
Accessory bones (lateral view)

thetic dystrophy especially in an immobilized patient. If reflex sympathetic dystrophy syndrome is diagnosed, appropriate therapy should begin immediately.

CALCANEAL FRACTURES

Calcaneal fractures can occur due to a fall from a height. Spine fractures are often associated with calcaneal fractures and should be ruled out. Essex, Lopresti, and Rowe have classified these fractures. A calcaneal fracture will almost always heal; however, some heal better than others. If the subtalar joint is involved most patients will develop arthritis, which can lead to long-term disability. Many articles have been written to help describe these fractures and dictate treatment modalities. The reader should be familiar with these articles if they treat calcaneal fractures. When immobilizing the lower extremity for prolonged periods caution and awareness of the possibility of phlebitis and deep venous thrombosis are necessary.

SUGGESTED READINGS

Rockwood CA, Jr, Green DP: Fractures in Adults 2nd Ed. JB Lippincott, Philadelphia, 1984

Scurran BL: Foot and Ankle Trauma. Churchill Livingstone, New York, 1989

6

CONGENITAL ANOMALIES

The most frequent complaints presented by the parent in the newborn and newly walking child are "my child's feet turn in," "my child's feet are flat," and "my child has an ingrown nail."

METATARSUS ADDUCTUS

Metatarsus adductus is when the metatarsals are turned inward toward the midline of the body causing the foot to be intoed (Fig. 23). This is usually characterized by a C-shaped outward border of the foot and a wider space between the great toe and second toe. The mother often complains that the child trips when walking. A pediatric lower extremity examination is necessary to determine whether the level of the deformity is in the foot or more proximal. A perinatal history is important; in determining the child's development include the following: lifting the head, rolling over, walking, talking, presence or absence of growing pains, and abnormal shoe wear. Familiarity with the developmental milestones is important in making use of this information. The perinatal history should be obtained for determination of whether or not the patient was full-term or premature, normal delivery or cesarean section, and what

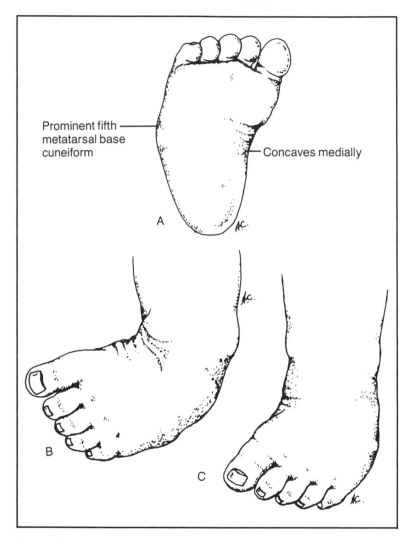

Prominent fifth
metatarsal base
cuneiform

Concaves medially

Figure 23
(A) Metatarus adductus. (B) Talipes equino varus. (C) Metadductus/
varus

the "Apgar" scores were at birth. The necessity of cesarean delivery can be due to stress on the child or mother during delivery, which can indicate the possibility of neurologic problems, and breach presentation can predispose to dislocated or dislocatable hips. Examination of the hip, knee, ankle, and subtalar joints are necessary. Developmental landmarks are important, especially, walking; age of walking is generally 9 to 16 months. If the patient is old enough to be wearing shoes, examination of the shoes is necessary. It is important to evaluate the shoe gear because children under the age of 2 may need 4 to 6 shoe size changes annually. A complete biomechanical or gait examination is important if the patient is ambulatory. If the hip, femur, knee and tibiofibular complexes are ruled out as being the etiology of the metatarsus adductus, and the deformity is flexible, usually the deformity can be successfully treated with manipulation and casting. This is best achieved when treatment is started before 1 year of age. Family history is extremely important, because of ontogenic expression of the deformity. When conservative therapy fails surgery is indicated to correct the deformity.

CLUBFOOT

The incidence of clubfoot is approximately 1:1,000 live births. This deformity should be recognized early. Treatment should begin as early as possible with serial casts. Despite appropriate conservative or surgical treatment, abnormal function and mild deformity may persist.

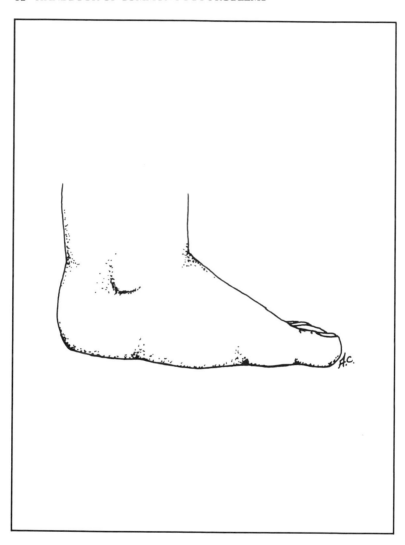

Figure 24
Flatfoot in a child

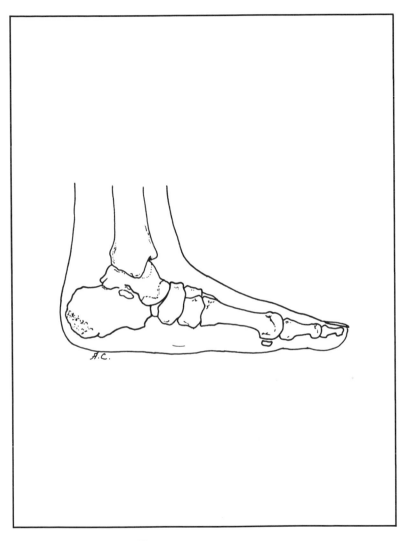

Figure 25
Flatfoot—note the plantarflexed position of the talus

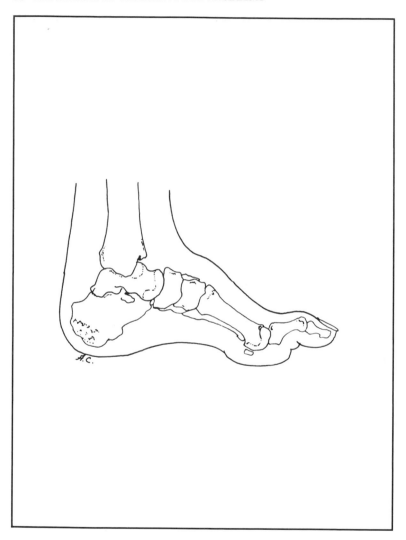

Figure 26
Cavus foot—note the increase in the angular relationships of the
calcaneous and metatarsal

FLATFOOT AND CAVUS FOOT

Frequently a child's foot is mistakenly called flat because of the fat pad within the arch in most young children. Development of the human begins in the central part of the body and extends distally. The feet and intrinsic musculature of the feet are among the last parts to develop. As the patient begins weight-bearing the appearance of the flatfoot often disappears. Cavus foot is a high arched foot and must be examined to determine the presence of a progressive neurologic disease versus a nonprogressive deformity. A progressive deformity with a possible neurologic etiology should be evaluated appropriately. The nonprogressive cavus foot is usually of hereditary origin; therefore, a family history is present (Figs. 24, 25, 26).

POLYDACTYLY

Polydactyly is not an emergency situation; however, evaluation for other abnormalities should take place. Definitive treatment should be delayed until it can be determined which digit is supernumery.

BRACHYMETATARSIA

Brachymetatarsia is a short metatarsal, most often the fourth. The etiology is usually congenital, however it can be acquired. Patients usually present at adolescence due to cosmesis or pain under an adjacent metatarsal head secondary to increased weight-bearing.

CONGENITAL INGROWN TOENAIL

The hallux nail is most frequently involved. The etiology is usually distal hypertrophy of the toe pulp and a broad flat nail.

SUGGESTED READINGS

Fixsen JA, Lloyd-Roberts GC: The Foot in Childhood. Churchill Livingstone, Edinburgh, 1989

Tachdjian M: The Child's Foot. WB Saunders, Philadelphia, 1985

Tax H: Podopediatrics. Williams & Wilkins, Baltimore, 1980

7

ACQUIRED COMPLAINTS

FOREFOOT PAIN

Corns

The most common digital cause of pain in the foot is a corn. This is a hyperkeratotic skin lesion seen on the dorsal, medial, lateral, or distal aspects of the toe. The etiology is irritation of the skin overlying a bony prominence. The corn is commonly seen; distally in the claw or mallet toe, dorsally in the claw or hammer toe, and medially or laterally in a toe with a bony prominence. These deformities are generally associated with poorly fit shoes and become more symptomatic with aging because of the the decreased mobility and flexibility of the foot. Biomechanical abnormalities generally can be related to the occurrence and progression of the claw toe and hammer toe. A mallet toe is a flexion contracture at the DIP with an associated corn on the dorsal aspect of the DIP joint or distal end of the toe. The second toe is most commonly affected. It is usually seen in a patient with a long second toe (Morton's toe). The etiology is shoe pressure causing retrograde force on the toe at the DIP joint. This happens because shoes are fitted to the great toe, not the longest toe, therefore if one toe is longer it will receive more pressure from the shoe (Figs. 27 and 28A).

The second most common forefoot complaint is pain in the ball of the foot. This is usually due to either plantar callosities, neuroma, or inflammatory arthropathy. When a foot has contracture of the digits at the MP joint, an increased force is placed on the metatarsal heads, a distal pull on the plantar fat pad, and a stretching of the plantar vital structures to the digits over the transverse metatarsal ligament. It is important to determine when the pain is worse and what relieves it. The contracted digit increases the force placed on the metatarsal head, the distal displacement of the fat pad decreases the cushioning of the plantar skin, and the stretching of the vital structures over the intermetatarsal ligament sets up an inflammatory response.

Neuroma

A neuroma is an inflammation or irritation of the common digital nerve as it passes between the metatarsal heads or over the deep transverse metatarsal ligament. The third interspace is most commonly affected; however, recent studies have shown that the second interspace is almost as common an area to be affected. This can be diagnosed clinically by eliciting pain when palpating the intermetatarsal space distal to the metatarsal heads in a dorsal/plantar direction. If the character of pain upon palpation is the same as when the patient walks, a clinical diagnosis will be confirmed. A neuroma can be differentiated from capsulitis, metatarsalgia, or inflammatory arthropathy by isolating the pain to the interspace and not the MP joint or plantar

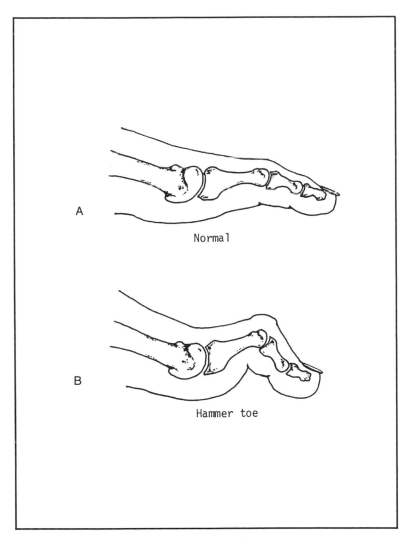

Figure 27
(*A*) Normal toe. (*B*) Hammer toe.

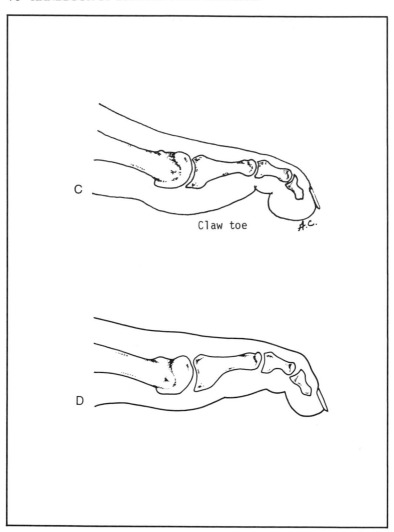

Figure 27
(C) Claw toe. (D) Mallet toe.

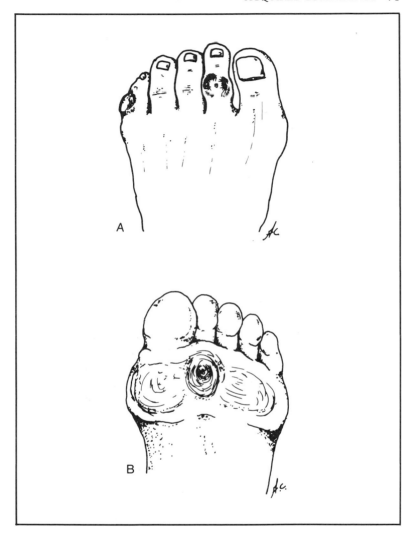

Figure 28
(A) Corns at the dorsum of the PIP joint. (B) Plantar callus

aspect of the metatarsal head. A selective diagnostic injection of a low volume of local anesthesia and steroid may help to differentiate these problems. Recent articles have illustrated the use of ultrasound imaging to identify the neuroma.

Callosities

With loss of the fat pad, prominence of the metatarsal heads, or long metatarsals, it is common to see calluses beneath the metatarsal heads. This is the foot type that will present with capsulitis or bursitis. A callus can be broad and flat usually due to shearing or rotational stresses. It can also be nucleated due to direct pressure. Occasionally, the patient will volunteer that the pain is worse on standing or walking and they will help differentiate the type of callus (Fig. 28B).

If the pain cannot be differentiated from the web or the metatarsal head, place the digit through a ROM at the DIP joint, PIP joint, and MP joint and note when the most pain occurs. Moving proximally, if the pain response is elicited with palpation of the neck and shaft of the metatarsal, a fracture is a likely cause. This diagnosis can be confirmed using radiographs or bone scans when necessary.

Capsulitis or bursitis

Capsulitis or bursitis is diagnosed when pain is elicited upon strict dorsal plantar palpation of the MP joint. Pain is usually worse on plantar palpation. Occasional edema may be noted.

The above are the most common problems of the forefoot excluding the first and fifth rays. The first and fifth rays both have independent ROMs and therefore tend to have similar problems.

Bunions

A tailor's bunion is prominence of the fifth metatarsal head dorsally and laterally. It is frequently associated with a varus rotated fifth toe. Presenting complaints are usually pain or difficulty fitting shoes. Clinically a prominent fifth metatarsal head with associated callus or bursitis is seen. After long-standing deformity with irritation, ganglions, neuromas, and synovial cysts have been associated with tailor's bunions. In the flexible splay foot it may be necessary to simulate weight-bearing or ask the patient to stand to notice the extent of the deformity. Treatment ranges from wider toe box shoes and pads to surgery if conservative therapy fails.

Hallux valgus is the lateral deviation of the hallux associated with a bunion on the medial side of the foot. The bunion prominence is the medial aspect fo the first metatarsal head that does not articulate with the hallux. The etiology of hallux valgus may include congenital, arthritis, hereditary (most common), biomechanical, and trauma. The deformity usually progresses due to the biomechanics of walking. Shoes as an etiology is a myth. Pain associated with the above deformities is of three origins: (1) irritation of the soft tissues by shoe gear, (2) irritation because of a degenerative process in the joint itself, (3) biomechancial limitation of motion.

Another type of bunion of the first MP joint is the dorsal bunion. It is often associated with hallux limitus or hallux rigidus. These are degenerative processes of

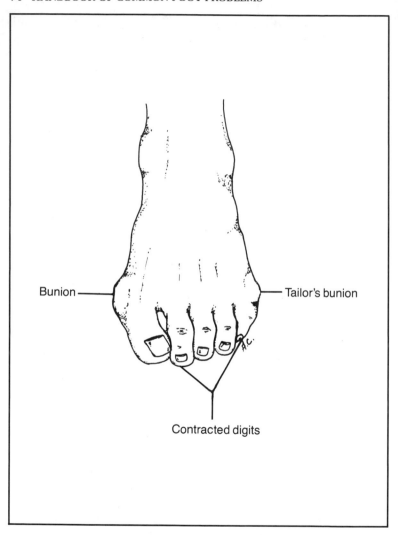

Figure 29
Common problems of the first and fifth rays

the first MP joint and will cause a limited range of motion of that joint. Frequently they are seen in a foot that has a long or dorsiflexed first metatarsal. Radiographs will help determine the cause and magnitude of the deformity (Fig. 29).

REARFOOT/MIDFOOT COMPLAINTS

The most common midfoot complaints are lumps or bumps in the midtarsal area of the foot with irritated overlying soft tissue. The most frequently encountered is the dorsal metatarsal-cuneiform exostosis. This is a bony prominence at the level of the first metatarsal cuneiform joint irritated by the vamp of the shoe. This deformity is usually seen in a flexible anterior cavus foot type with a hypermobile or flexible first metatarsal joint. The increased motion of the metatarsal causes increased retrograde forces at the metatarsal cuneiform joint causing increased bone formation (Wolfe's law). Chronic irritation by shoe gear can lead to ganglions or a compression neuropathy of the deep peroneal nerve. Surgery is the best treatment followed with orthotics to control abnormal motion.

The most common complaint in the rear part of the foot is plantar fasciitis or heel spur syndrome. This must be differentiated from heel neuroma, posterior tibial tendon strain, fracture of the calcaneus, and systemic causes.

To differentiate the complaints of pain on the plantar aspect of the rearfoot it is important to determine the nature of the pain and its characteristics. Pain upon palpation at the origin of the plantar fascia along the medial plantar aspect of the calcaneus is consistent with plantar fasciitis. The pain is generally worse upon initial weight-bearing in the morning, improves with activity, and after resting and resumption of activity pain will increase again. Radiographs often reveal a spur at the insertion of the plantar fasciia; however, this is not always the etiology. All spurs do not cause heel pain and all heel pain is not caused by spurs. On the other hand, if pain is produced by palpation along the course of the posterior tibial tendon as it circles the medial aspect of the ankle and inserts into the navicular area of the medial plantar of the foot, a reasonable certainty exists that there is some type of irritation of the posterior tibial tendon. This may be confirmed by resisting the patient's plantarflexion-inversion or by asking the patient to toe-walk and reproducing the symptoms. Acute rupture of the posterior tibial tendon is associated with acute flattening of the longitudinal arch of the foot. Pain that can be reproduced by percussing the posterior tibial nerve at the level of the ankle will more than likely be tarsal tunnel syndrome. Medial calcaneal nerve entrapment syndrome (heel neuroma) can be present as a separate or a co-existing problem with plantar fasciitis. Radiating or burning pain localized to the plantar medial aspect of the heel in conjunction with a palpable mass plantar and proximal to the porta pedis is consistent with heel neuroma. If there is radiation of pain to the plantar heel, entrapment of the calcaneal branch of the posterior tibial nerve is likely. If patients relate a similar type of pain, but that the pain is worse the more they bear weight, then plantar fasciitis can often be ruled out and other causes must be considered. Radiographs are useful to determine the etiology.

Another common rearfoot complaint is pain at the

posterior aspect of the heel. A differential diagnosis should include Achilles tendonitis, calcaneal bursitis, retrocalcaneal bursitis, or Haglund's deformity. To differentiate these four, localization of the pain is of utmost importance. Pain directly posterior to the bony prominence at the insertion of the Achilles tendon is retrocalcaneal bursitis secondary to Haglund's deformity. Whereas pain anterior to the Achilles tendon is calcaneal bursitis. If pain is elicited upon palpation of the Achilles tendon or movement of the tendon, this is indicative of Achilles tendonitis. A very common radiographic finding is bony spurring at the insertion of the Achilles tendon. The spur is usually not the etiology of pain and seldom requires removal.

Pain localized to the posterior aspect of the calcaneus in adolescent children (9- to 12-year-old girls and 9- to 15-year-old boys) is consistent with a diagnosis of calcaneal apophysitis. The calcaneus has a secondary growth center that ossifies to its body at age 12 in girls and age 14 to 15 in boys. This growth center becomes inflamed in patients that are very active in sports. Treatment consists of immobilization and orthotics. Often casts are needed to decrease activity to allow healing. In growing children, usually during the adolescent growth spurt, posterior heel pain can be related to calcaneal apophysitis. It is often associated with increased activity, stiff shoes, and activity on hard unforgiving surfaces.

Acute rupture of the Achilles tendon will present in the middle-aged athlete with pain and inability to plantarflex the foot at the ankle or walk upstairs. Oftentimes palpation of the Achilles tendon will show a gap between the ends of the tendon. Partial ruptures will show weakness, pain, and increased pain when attempting toe raises.

SUGGESTED READINGS

Jahss MA: The Foot. WB Saunders, Philadelphia, 1982

McGlamry ED: Comprehensive Textbook of Foot Surgery. Williams & Wilkins, Baltimore, 1987

8

LOCAL MANIFESTATIONS OF SYSTEMIC DISEASE

It was once said that the foot is a mirror of systemic disease. The initial clinical presentation of diseases including diabetes mellitus, rheumatoid arthritis, gout, and vascular disease often begins in the foot. This chapter discusses the pedal manifestation of diabetes mellitus and rheumatoid arthritis.

Foot complaints are commonly the first presenting signs of diabetes mellitus. The etiology of these complaints are predominantly vascular and neurologic processes; however, the dermatologic and musculoskeletal systems may be involved. Therefore, from an evaluation perspective these complaints are divided into neuropathic, ischemic, dermatologic, and musculoskeletal complaints. Patients can present with either type of complaint, or they may present together.

NEUROPATHIC FOOT

The initial clinical signs of neuropathy include hemorrhage beneath a nail or within a callus in a patient with no history of trauma, hyperhidrosis, unexplained bruising, difficulty fitting shoes, or ulceration. This foot is warm and hyperemic. Paresthesia type symptoms, i.e., burning, numbness, tingling, and cramps due to neuropathy should be differentiated from symptoms of peripheral vascular disease. Paresthesias due to neuropathy are constant and prevent the patient from sleeping, although they may be temporarily alleviated by increased activity; whereas vascular "rest" pain is usually worse at night and will awaken a sleeping patient. Relief is achieved predictably by placing the limb in a position of dependency and getting out of bed and sitting in a chair. The diagnosis can be confirmed by a lower extremity neurologic examination that includes patellar and Achilles deep tendon reflexes, which are decreased or absent, proprioception, sharp-dull sensation, vibratory sensation, and hot and cold temperature sensations, which are slowed or absent. Semmes-Weinstein monofilaments should also be applied to the digits and foot to assess protective threshold. The clinician must be aware that the answers to the above examinations are yes or no and that the response time for those answers is also important, i.e., if a patient responds yes but there is a time delay of 5 seconds this answer is significantly different from the patient who answers yes almost immediately. It is also important to repeat this clinical examination over time to establish a baseline of findings for the patient as well as monitor the progression of the neurologic changes. Nerve conduction velocity can be used to further document neuropathy and to give a quantifiable measure of progression of the neuropathy. Later signs of neuropathy are hypertrophic callus with ulcers beneath the callus, intrinsic minus foot, which causes hammer toes, plantarly prominent metatarsal heads, with abnormal weight-bearing intrinsic muscle wasting, foot drop, and ulceration. Neuroarthropathy changes of the foot may include cardinal signs of inflammation, heat, or increased edema, without infection or known history of trauma. Radiographic findings of collapse and abduction of the longitudinal arch, stress fractures, hypertrophy of the cortices of the metatarsals, and occasionally disappearance of the bony structure of the metatarsals due to osteolysis are consistent with neuroarthropathy. These same signs can be seen with alcohol-related neuropathy. The clinician should be observant for these clinical and radiographic changes and their relationship to clinical symptomatology. These ulcers are pathognomic and show hyperkeratotic borders, vascular base with granulation tissue and smooth contours. The ulcers are also related to a bony prominence. The foot is usually warm, with palpable pulses, hair growth, supple skin, and venous distention. The ulcers are seen at the first and fifth metatarsal heads and are associated with bony deformities and mechanical irritation often presenting beneath a callus, which has been present for a long time but has not been symptomatic because of the neuropathy. Often these ulcers become infected and the underlying bone becomes involved because the patient does not realize that the ulcer is present (Fig.30).

ISCHEMIC FOOT

The patient with an ischemic foot classically presents with a cold foot with atrophic skin, absence of hair growth, dystrophic nails, delayed capillary refill time, and a history of noctural pain and/or intermittent claudication. Clinically the foot exhibits all the signs and

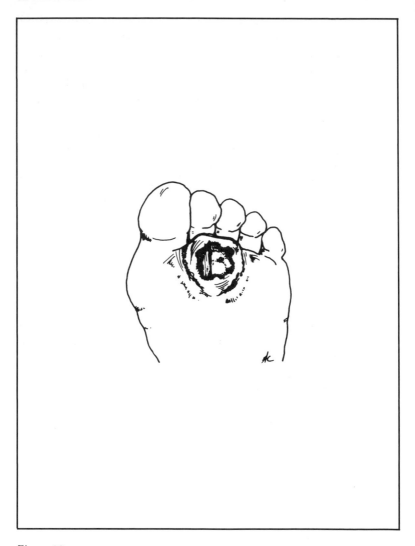

Figure 30.
Neurotrophic ulcer—note the hypertrophic borders and granular base

symptoms of vascular disease in the diabetic foot and leg including erythema on dependency and pallor on elevation, nonpalpable dorsalis pedis and posterior tibial pulses, decreased pulsatility on Doppler examination, sluggish capillary refill time, loss of hair, dry scaling skin, hypertrophic, dystrophic nails, or clubbing of nails.

When the history reveals rapid increase in symptoms or signs, it is necessary to perform a segmental Doppler examination to rule out an acute occlusion that most likely occurs at the trifurcation of the popliteal artery just distal to the popliteal fossa. A timely vascular consultation for consideration of arterial bypass grafting may save the patient's limb. Ischemic ulcers are painful with pale, yellow-gray, necrotic, nonbleeding bases. They are covered with fibrous eschar with jagged edges and hypotrophic borders. The ulcers are generally located on the digits or over a bony prominence and have a necrotic fibrous base. Many of the lesions progress to gangrene of the digits or a portion of the forefoot. Revascularization is the key to healing this lesion and to prevent amputation (Figs. 31 and 32).

RHEUMATOID FOOT

Rheumatoid foot is a form of arthritis that primarily affects the MP joints; however, all joints can be involved. The most common problems include hallux valgus, hammer toes with dislocation at the MP joints, fibular deviation of the toes, intrinsic muscular atrophy, posterior tibial tendonitis, talonavicular strain, and rheumatoid nodules overlying bony prominences. Appropriate shoes and shoe gear modifications can be ade-

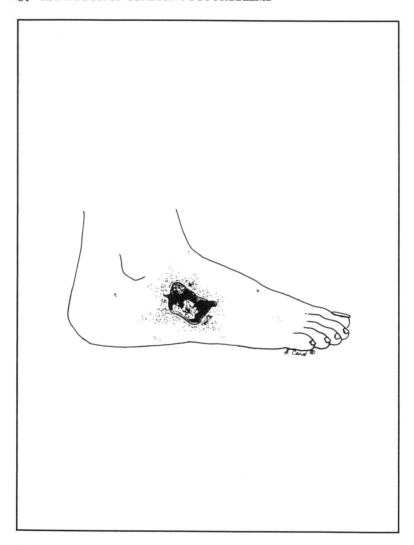

Figure 31
Ischemic ulcer—note the hypotrophic borders and eschar base

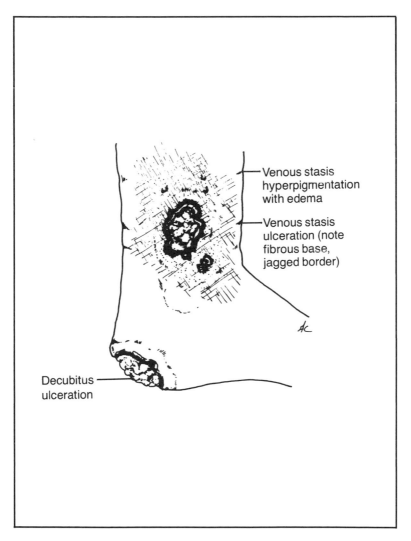

Figure 32
Vasculitic and decubitus ulcer

quate treatment for patients with active systemic disease. However, when the pain or deformity cannot be managed conservatively, surgical intervention is indicated. Surgery in the rheumatoid foot alleviates pain, corrects the deformity, and improves function.

It is important to discuss this patient with the physician who is managing the patient due to the systemic manifestions of the disease and the medications used to treat this disease. The acutely inflamed joint should be reviewed. The differential diagnosis for the patient who presents with an acutely swollen, warm, and erythematous MP joint of the first digit should include, gout, pseudo-gout, infection, trauma, pigmented villanodular synovitis, and early rheumatoid arthritis. Trauma can usually be ruled out by history, except for a stress fracture, infection by a normal white blood count, and the remaining diagnoses by a joint aspirate and analysis of the joint fluid. A stress fracture is an incomplete fracture that usually presents in a patient with acute onset of pain and swelling of the foot with no history of trauma. Often the patient will give a history of increased activity that usually predisposes the bone to more stress, therefore, causing the problem.

DERMATOLOGIC LESIONS

Dermatologic lesions are divided into primary and secondary lesions. To arrive at a differential diagnosis it is important clinically to describe the lesion and place it into either one of the primary or secondary lesion categories. Once this is done the differential diagnosis can be determined from the nature of the lesion. For example, a primary problem would provide a differential of tinea pedis, psoriasis, dyshidrotic eczema and pityriasis rosea, or pityriasis rubra pilaris, versus a lichonfied or excoriation which may suggest scabies.

SUGGESTED READINGS

Boulton AJM, Connor H, Ward JD: The Foot in Diabetes. J Wiley & Sons, New York, 1987

Harkless LB, Dennis KJ: The diabetic foot. Clin Podiatr Med Surg 4:2, 1987

Levin ME, O'Neal LW: The Diabetic Foot. CV Mosby, St. Louis. 1988

Pack LG: Acute adult inflammatory pedal arthritis: a practical guide to diagnosis, J AM Podiatr Assoc 66(9): 663, 1976

Jay RM: Current Therapy in Podiatric Surgery. BC Decker, Philadelphia, 1989

9

SPORTS INJURIES

The foot and the ankle are the most commonly injured body parts in sports.

RUNNING INJURIES

Injuries incurred during running sports can be divided into two basic groups: overuse injuries and ballistic injuries.

Overuse injuries

The most common injuries are the overuse type injuries where the patient did not reduce their activities in the presence of warning signs such as pain. Common overuse injuries include plantar fasciitis, MP joint bursitis, capsulitis, peroneal tendonitis, shin splints, and sesamoiditis.

Shin splints

Shin splints or anterior or posterior tibial tendonitis are commonly seen in athletes who have changed their work-out habits. Those who exercise over hilly terrain are more susceptible. With shin splints, the differentials, stress fractures of the tibia and compartment syndrome should be ruled out in recalcitrant cases. A stress fracture will be a well-localized point tenderness readily confirmed with a bone scan. Compartment syndromes, of which the deep posterior compartment is most commonly involved can be ruled out by normal sensation in the first web space of the involved foot and normal extensor-flexor function of the extensor hallucis longus.

Tendonitis/bursitis

Tendonitis and bursitis often go hand in hand. They can occur almost anywhere there are tendons or bursae on the foot. The most common locations are those of the Achilles tendon and Achilles bursae. They can be differentiated by its proximity to the insertion of the Achilles tendon. Palpation of the Achilles tendon proximal to its insertion with a pain response will support the clinical diagnosis of Achilles tendonitis. In a middle-aged patient, if palpation shows a definite dell or space between the longitudinal fibers of the tendon, a rupture or partial rupture should be considered. Retrocalcaneal bursitis, infracalcaneal bursitis, and posterior Achilles bursitis can be differentiated by palpation and localizing the area of maximum pain—either posterior or superficial to the tendon, immediately deep to the tendon, or at the insertion of the tendon to the calcaneus. Posterior tibial tendonitis is often seen in patients with excessive pronation lacking a supportive heal counter or arch support.

Stress fractures

Stress fractures most often occur in the lesser metatarsals of the forefoot. Commonly called "march" fractures, they are seen in military recruits and in people whose athletic activity is performed on the ball of the foot—aerobics, running, etc. Radiographs will usually show minimal periosteal reaction until approximately 2 to 3 weeks after the injury. Calcaneal stress fractures usually also occur in adults; children 10 to 14 years of age often present with heel pain which can be related to activity. Radiographs will often exhibit an open epiphysis and without other signs a presumptive diagnosis of calcaneal apophysis can be made. Often side-to-side pressure on the body of the calcaneus will elicit a pain response and this will usually rule out heel spur syndrome or plantar fasciitis.

Ballistic injuries

Ballistic movements are movements used when changing direction and speed quickly. These injuries occur in court sports, sprints, baseball, and softball. The most common injuries are sprains, strains, and muscle ruptures.

Ankle sprains

Ankle sprains are commonly seen in sports played on uneven terrain or in sports with a lot of vertical changes (i.e. basketball, volleyball). In the vertical sports, the most common injury is the inversion ankle sprain. Plantarflexing the foot at the ankle places stretch on the anterior talofibular ligament and when the foot inverts this will injure this ligament (See Figs. 16, 17, 18). It is important to determine the sequence of injury to help determine the extent of injury. Eversion ankle injuries to the deltoid ligament are far less common and more serious, and are beyond the scope of this book. Basically, an injury to the medial ankle indicates a much more severe injury.

CHILDHOOD ANKLE INJURIES

In all ankle injuries of younger children it is more likely to see avulsion fractures than ligamentous injury. Therefore, Salter type fractures should be considered with contralateral examination and radiographic evaluation used to determine the extent of injury.

MUSCLE STRAINS AND RUPTURES

Poor warm-up and training techniques, or overuse in a pronated or flatfoot are often the cause of muscle sprains and ruptures. This injury is associated with severe pain. The three most common muscles involved are the gastrocnemius soleus complex, the posterior tibial muscle, and the peroneal muscles. If overuse is the etiology, training adjustments and an orthotic will usually alleviate the symptoms.

The *gastroctendo-Achilles* injury is associated with painful or weak plantarflexion of the foot at the ankle. Often palpation of the Achilles tendon just proximal to its insertion will elicit a pain response. If the patient lies prone on the examining table with the knee of the affected leg flexed at 90 degrees, an intact tendon will be illustrated when the foot plantarflexes after squeezing the calf. Failure to elicit plantarflexion suggests a complete tear of this complex. Occasionally this injury can be from the proximal insertion of the gastrocnemius muscle and therefore the posterior knee should always be examined.

The *posterior tibial* injury is most often seen in overweight individuals who wear improper shoe gear. Pain is localized to the area immediately posterior to the medial malleolus. The function of the posterior tibial muscle can be assessed by having the patient push the inside of their foot against your hand while holding the foot in a plantarflexed position. If the patient is unable to perform this maneuver or this motion creates discomfort for the patient the posterior tibial tendon is involved.

The *peroneal muscles* are commonly injured in the lateral ankle injury. The peroneus brevis tendon can be palpated from the base of the fifth metatarsal along its course posterior to the lateral malleolus. The peroneus longus tendon can be palpated from the plantar aspect of the cuboid to the lateral malleolus (where it lies posterior to the peroneus brevis). Occasionally, a subluxing peroneal tendon can be noted when the patient ambulates, or by having the examiner resist external rotation motion of the foot on the leg

SUGGESTED READINGS

Subotnick SI: Sports Medicine of the Lower Extremity. Churchill Livingstone, New York, 1989

Sports Medicine. Clin Podiatr Med Surg 3 (4), 1986

10

BIOMECHANICS

The foot serves two main functions; one as a mobile adapter and the other as a rigid lever for propulsion. These two functions are time specific, i.e., when the foot spends too much time as a mobile adapter it cannot spend enough time as a rigid lever and vice-versa. Biomechanics of the foot are used to determine how well the foot performs these functions. Excessive motion or lack of motion will cause the various deformities discussed elsewhere in this book.

This equates to excessive pronation = too much time as a mobile adapter or inadequate pronation = too much time as a rigid lever.

PRONATION

Pronation is the function of the foot as a mobile adapter, which is necessary to adjust to varied terrains and unexpected situations. The second pronation function is as a shock absorber. As the foot pronates, the posterior tibial and anterior tibial muscles function to slow the weight transfer and decrease the shock going up the leg. Excessive pronation can be due to increased activity, increased weight, or poor structural support and cause the muscles to work harder to maintain stance for propulsion.

SUPINATION

Supination is the function of the foot changing from a mobile adapter to a rigid lever for propulsion. Often the foot is in a supinated position as in the cavus foot or in a foot with tibial varum. The patients will use their entire pronatory motion in attempts to keep the foot in contact with the ground. These patients then lose their shock absorption ability and will often exhibit signs of poor shock absorption.

JOINT MOTIONS

Ankle joint

The primary motion at the ankle joint is dorsiflexion and plantarflexion in the sagittal plane. As Figure 3 illustrates, 10 degrees of dorsiflexion and 45 degrees of plantarflexion are necessary for normal gait. The ankle joint is often injured in the patient with a cavus foot type due to the long moment arm and the imbalance created by the inverted heel.

Subtalar joint

The primary motion at the subtalar joint is inversion and eversion in the frontal plane, even though the subtalar joint has triplane motion (see Figs. 4 and 5). The total amount of motion is variable; however, there is approximately twice as much inversion needed as eversion. This is measured by visualizing the bisection of the lower leg and the bisection of the calcaneus while everting the calcaneus maximally and then inverting the calcaneus maximally.

Calcaneal stance position

This measurement is important to determine if a patient is using their entire eversion motion during stance. This is determined by comparing the maximum eversion in degrees with the calcaneal stance position in degrees. This is measured by the angle created by the bisection of the lower leg and calcaneus in stance.

Midtarsal joint

The midtarsal joint's function is directly related to the function of the subtalar joint (see Fig. 5). When the subtalar joint is pronated, the midtarsal joint unlocks, thus allowing the foot to adapt to the terrain. When the subtalar joint is supinated the midtarsal joint locks, allowing the foot to function as a rigid lever. Again, if pronation time is excessive the midtarsal joint will remain unlocked too long, a flacid forefoot will result and muscular function will be necessary to attempt to change the foot to a rigid lever. This is often the cause of clawing the toes and the formation of bunions and cramping of the lower leg.

If the phase of pronation is too short, the foot functions in a supinated attitude. This then causes a large amount of shock to be transmitted up the leg. In this case the muscles function to slow the shock and attempt to bring the locked midtarsal joint to the ground slower. This often will cause the contractures usually in a sagittal plane as seen in the cavus foot.

First MP joints

The first ray is the primary propulsive lever of the forefoot. The first ray is stabilized by the function of the peroneus longus muscle. Again, if pronation time is excessive the peroneus longus will lose its fulcrum of support and will not be able to help in the stabilization of the first ray. If pronation is inadequate the peroneus longus will plantarflex the first ray in an effort to bring the first ray to the ground.

The first MP joint is actually three joints, the hallux, first metatarsal, and the two sesamoids and the first metatarsal head. The sesamoid's purpose is to serve as a fulcrum to provide added strength to the flexor hallucis brevis for stabilizing the great toe for propulsion. Normal motion of the hallux at the first MP joint is 20 degrees of plantarflexion and approximately 90 degrees of dorsiflexion. Less than 40 degrees of dorsiflexion is considered hallux limitus. This motion is dependent on the ability of the first ray to plantarflex. A functional limitus is seen where the first ray is not allowed to plantarflex thus limiting the available dorsiflexion at the first metatarsal phalangeal joint.

IP joints

The main purpose of the IP joints is to allow muscle function to stabilize the foot against the ground (see Fig. 6). In rigid soled shoes or hard level surfaces this proprioceptive function is not necessary.

SUGGESTED READINGS

Root ML, Weed JH, Orien WP: Normal and Abnormal Function of the Foot. Vols. I & II, 1977

Yale J: Podiatric Medicine. William & Wilkins, Baltimore, 1987

Applied biomechanics. Clin Podiatr Med Surg. 5(3), 1988

INDEX

Page numbers followed by f indicate figures; those followed by t indicate tables.